Lucynara Gomes Lima Tambon
Marcos Almeida Matos

Predisposing factors for open fracture infection and score

Lucynara Gomes Lima Tambon
Marcos Almeida Matos

Predisposing factors for open fracture infection and score

'Predisposing factors for infection in patients with open fractures and creation of a score'

ScienciaScripts

Imprint
Any brand names and product names mentioned in this book are subject to trademark, brand or patent protection and are trademarks or registered trademarks of their respective holders. The use of brand names, product names, common names, trade names, product descriptions etc. even without a particular marking in this work is in no way to be construed to mean that such names may be regarded as unrestricted in respect of trademark and brand protection legislation and could thus be used by anyone.

Cover image: www.ingimage.com

This book is a translation from the original published under ISBN 978-613-9-66912-7.

Publisher:
Sciencia Scripts
is a trademark of
Dodo Books Indian Ocean Ltd. and OmniScriptum S.R.L publishing group

120 High Road, East Finchley, London, N2 9ED, United Kingdom
Str. Armeneasca 28/1, office 1, Chisinau MD-2012, Republic of Moldova, Europe
Printed at: see last page
ISBN: 978-620-8-11218-9

Special thanks

To my dear parents, Ulisses Barros Lima and Elezenita Gomes Lima, I express my eternal gratitude for their love, their example, for being by my side and for believing in my dreams. I'm looking for words and I can't find them to show how sorry I am today, Dad, for the hours I wasn't able to enjoy by your side, because of this process, for trying to build something that you believed was important for our lives. It was very difficult to overcome the loss of you during this construction, at a time when your presence would have been very important to me. I didn't have time to show you the result of this in life, but I know that where you are you will understand and be proud of me, you will see that I learnt the life lesson you left me: to fight with dignity, character, humility and persistence in pursuit of a dream. To my beloved mother, I thank you for being an example of a mother, a woman, a friend, a warrior, for your strength, your prayers and your incomparable love.

To my husband, Mareei Tambon Nascimento, and my son Daniel L. T. Nascimento, I thank you for your love, your support, for understanding my absences, for understanding my nervous states, for encouraging me to keep going, for making me believe that I would be able to overcome this stage. To my son, for his sensitivity in understanding my moments of despair, tiredness and neediness, for his affection, massages, compliments and for proving to be my greatest friend.

I would like to thank my sisters, Luciene Lima de Andrade, Lucy Lima Muniz Ferreira and Luciana Gomes Lima, for their love, affection, support and encouragement, for often covering my absences by looking after my son, my parents and my husband.

To my brothers-in-law Carlos Alberto de Andrade and Edilson Muniz Ferreira, and my nephews Gabriel Andrade, Pedro Muniz and Vitoria Muniz, I thank you for your love, your companionship, your hours of distraction and joy, for distracting my husband, my son and my parents during my absences to do this work.

To my family in general, especially my aunts Fza, Ezeni, Loi, Lene, Lurdes, and my cousins, but especially to Sissi, Marli, Suzi and Márcia Santos, for their encouragement, for believing in me, for their prayers and above all for the great love they have given me, which strengthens me.

I have a great wealth, which is my family. I can't thank them all specifically, as it would make a book, but those who have been most present in some way.

I thank God immensely for being present in my life and for having this wonderful family that I love!

TEAM:

Lucynara Gomes Lima, master's student.

Marcos Almeida Matos, supervisor.

Rômulo Neves Castro Filho, participant in the data collection.

Julia Milena N. do Nascimento, participant in the data collection.

Thank you

To say thank you is to remember all the moments when this work was being done, to remember all the people who contributed to this challenge. It's recognising the special people in our lives, those who have helped us to follow the best path. Those who helped overcome the difficulties, the lost nights, the hours of tiredness, the moments of anguish, who didn't let me lose heart, who encouraged me to keep fighting, who made me realise that the time had come to turn obstacles into achievements.

Firstly, I thank God, my guide, my light, who knows deep down how I feel about life, my weaknesses, my dreams and who shows me how to overcome the difficulties along the way.

To my colleagues in the master's programme, especially Cristiane Gusmão and Ana Shirlei for their affection, support, criticism and sincere friendship, and to the rest of my colleagues who shared moments of learning, relaxation and friendship during this process.

To my colleague Liliam Brito, for her friendship and for her collaboration in the construction of this work.

To Antoniel Barros, professor of statistics at Faculdade D. Pedro II, where we are work colleagues, a great friend, who helped me to better understand the analyses of my research.

To the masters, in particular, for their dedication, wisdom, for showing me the way and for helping me grow on this journey:

To my former teachers at that institution, now coordinator Kátia Sá and Professor Abrahão Baptista, for their ideas on how to construct the work, for their criticism, support and affection.

To Professor Luis Cláudio Corrêa for teaching me statistics, for his gift of making such a complex subject easier to learn by making it simpler.

To Professor Mário Rocha, Carlos Alfredo Marcílio de Souza and Constança Cruz, for the moments of pleasurable learning with discussions that enriched my master's degree and my life.

To Professor Bruno Gil, for the brilliant ethics lessons and the unique moments with someone so captivating, charismatic and competent, who made the lessons flow in a light and constructive way.

To the professors, Ana Marice Ladeia and Professor Arménio Gimarães, for their criticism, example of discipline and wisdom.

3

To my friends, for realising that in this process I needed seclusion and to get away from their good company.

In particular, I would like to thank a great friend, Regina Sturaro, to whom I owe a lot for her unconditional love, support, prayers and for making me believe that I would succeed at the end of this work.

To my patients, for their understanding, for often leaving them without appointments to prioritise stages that would be necessary in the construction of this dissertation, and to the patients who took part in this research by making their data available.

To the managers of the Roberto Santos General Hospital for allowing this work to be carried out there.

To the staff of the Bahiana School of Medicine and Public Health for their warm help on this journey.

For me, giving thanks means recognising the value of each person, it means realising that we need each other for our projects to come to fruition. We need the affection, the support, the criticism, the understanding, the examples, the encouragement of people with whom we will have the pleasure of celebrating the joy of having done our duty, of having won a victory.

"For a dream dreamt alone is a dream, and a dream dreamt together is reality."

Special thanks

I would like to say a huge thank you to my advisor Dr Marcos Almeida Matos for his hours of dedication, patience, understanding, wisdom, criticism, for believing in me and helping me to build something that has a lot of value in my life.

SUMMARY

SUMMARY

Introduction: The main objectives of orthopaedic treatment for open fractures are the prevention of infection, stabilisation of the bone lesion and restoration of limb function. Preventing infection, however, is the main measure for achieving the other objectives. **Objective.** To identify the risk factors associated with infection in patients affected by open fractures, using the strength of association of these factors to propose a score that enables risk stratification in initial care. **Patients and Methods.** A retrospective analysis was carried out. The study included all patients who underwent open fracture treatment at the Roberto Santos General Hospital (HGRS), Salvador, Bahia, Brazil, from March to December 2009. Patients with open fractures of the axial skeleton (face, skull, thorax), children under 8 years of age and those who did not remain in the hospital for at least one day after the initial procedure, either due to death or transfer, were excluded from the study. Patients whose medical records did not contain the information sought in the study were also excluded. Clinical and demographic data was collected and the results were divided into two groups: patients with and without infection. Both groups were assessed for associated factors that could lead to infection. **Results.** 122 patients were studied. The overall infection rate was 25.4 per cent. Patients from inland areas were more likely to develop an infection (61.3%), as were those with an exposure time of more than 24 hours (average of 30.3 *hours, p* = 0.007). Fractures classified as Gustillo III had a higher chance of infection (74.2%, p = 0.042), especially IIIB (41.9%). Fractures classified as Tscheme II and III had a higher chance of infection (48.4% and 25.8%, p = 0.001). **Conclusions.** It was possible to identify that exposure time, fracture classification according to Gustillo and injury classification according to Tscheme are associated with the outcome of infection in open fractures. It was also possible to create a risk score to predict infection in this type of fracture (ERI), which can be used in initial patient care, with a sensitivity of 0.840, specificity of 0.544, cut-off point of 6.5 and area under *the* curve of 0.709 (p = 0.002).

Keywords: open fracture; infection; treatment; trauma; score.

CHAPTER 1

INTRODUCTION

The main objectives of orthopaedic treatment for open fractures are the prevention of infection, stabilisation of the bone lesion and restoration of limb function. Preventing infection, however, is the main measure for achieving the other objectives[1,2,3].

A post-traumatic bone infection (osteomyelitis) is a devastating event that will certainly compromise the patient's treatment and rehabilitation. In addition, post-traumatic osteomyelitis increases the cost and duration of treatment too much, causing human and social damage that can jeopardise the quality of life and functional independence of individuals[4].

Surgical cleaning with debridement as early as possible, preferably before six hours after the injury, combined with immediate stabilisation are the most effective measures for preventing infection in the treatment of open fractures[1,2,3]. Although these measures are fundamental, several other clinical and socio-environmental factors also contribute significantly to the onset of post-traumatic osteomyelitis. The main risk factors associated with infection include the energy involved in the trauma, the extent of the injury and soft tissue devitalisation, the severity of the bone damage, the degree of local contamination, the delay in instituting initial treatment and the patient's immune status[5,6,7].

The identification of risk factors predictive of infection in the initial clinical assessment of patients with open fractures should therefore be a crucial stage in orthopaedic treatment. Immediate recognition of these indicators could result in more effective therapeutic measures being taken as early and appropriately as possible. Thus, from the first moment of treatment, risk stratification would help the orthopaedic surgeon choose the best course of action for patients at high risk of developing infection.

Despite recognising the importance of clinical and socio-environmental risk factors in the treatment and prognosis of open fractures, most studies on this subject have focused on surgical aspects[8,9,10,11,12]. This study aims to identify the risk factors associated with infection in patients with open fractures, using the strength of association of these factors to propose a score that enables risk stratification in initial care.

CHAPTER 2

LITERATURE REVIEW

2.1 INTRODUCTION

The current era has been marked by a high rate of injuries, and several factors have contributed to this, such as car accidents, accidents at work, falls, cave-ins, burns, accidents with bladed weapons and firearms[13] . This is mainly due to the increased participation of individuals in high-speed traffic, complex industries, competitive and recreational sports, in short, technological advances and the lifestyle of modern individuals. This increase in accidents is growing year on year, as is their severity. Suffice to say that currently around a third of the beds in hospital surgical wards are occupied by injured patients. This is what we can call the age of injury or the age of trauma, as Salter points out[13] . Of these significant injuries, at least two thirds involve the musculoskeletal system: fractures, dislocations and soft tissue injuries. Injuries have therefore increased in frequency and importance.

[aa]Trauma in Western countries is the 3rd leading cause of death, after cardiovascular disease and cancer, and in people under 45 years of age it is the 1st leading cause of death. It mainly affects the economically active population, with costly social consequences. If the patient survives the trauma, there may be permanent and irreversible sequelae, with adverse human and economic consequences for the patient and their family[14] .

Salter[13] emphasises that some of these injuries may not be fatal, but they are important because most of them cause a lot of physical and mental suffering and loss of time for the victim. Of these injuries, fractures will be the most relevant to this study, as they represent a public health problem with a high incidence and socio-economic cost, and are an important cause of morbidity and mortality, with the morbidity rate being higher than the mortality rate.

2.2 DEFINITIONS

A **bone fracture** is a situation in which there is a loss of bone continuity, usually with the separation of a bone into two or more fragments after trauma[15] . Their severity can vary greatly; some fractures resolve spontaneously without being diagnosed, while others are life-threatening and are medical emergencies.

When we refer to a fracture, we initially think of an injury characterised by the loss of continuity of a bone segment. But when we analyse the injury further, we realise that the fracture should actually be called a **fracture complex,** as it can be a combination of local soft tissue injuries and the bone injury itself. The soft tissue lesions are just as important in the assessment, treatment and prognosis of fracture healing as the bone lesions, as they represent the important factor of vascularisation and, ultimately, the biological factor of healing.

2.3 FRACTURE CLASSIFICATION

Classically, we divide fractures into two distinct types: closed fractures and open fractures:

CLOSED FRACTURES: these are fractures in which there is no rupture of the skin and consequently no communication between the fracture site and the external environment[15] . They are generally treated orthopaedically, but in certain cases require immediate surgical treatment when there is vascular damage, nerve compression, fracture instability and in polytraumatised patients (due to the need for early mobilisation). These fractures have a better prognosis for treatment because they are less likely to be infected.

EXPOSED **FRACTURES:** an exposed fracture is one in which there is a break in the skin and underlying soft tissues directly communicating the fracture site with the outside environment or to contaminated cavities such as the mouth, digestive tract, airways, vagina and anus[16][17] . Thus, a fracture of the pelvis that is exposed through the vaginal wall is considered an open fracture and is particularly serious due to the richness of the local bacterial flora. Open fractures generally involve high energy to occur, with concomitant injury to the soft tissues, which favours infection by germs, as well as hindering healing.

Open fractures, in particular, are subject to infection and delayed healing, which are the main problems associated with them.

The seriousness of open fractures has been well understood since ancient times. Hippocratic physicians recognised that the size of the wound, the stability of the fracture and the proximity of neurovascular structures influenced the final outcome of these serious injuries[18] . It is important to be familiar with the various traumatic injuries, as well as the emergency measures that should be taken in the case of an injured person with an open fracture.

Therefore, the classification of open fractures is essential because it allows for the comparison of results in scientific publications, and is even more important because it allows surgeons to follow guidelines regarding the prognosis of these fractures and provides guidance on treatment methods, allowing for the incidence of complications by preventing errors[19] .

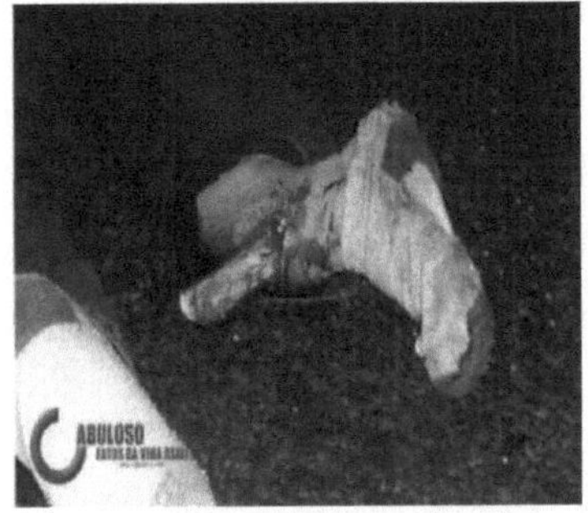
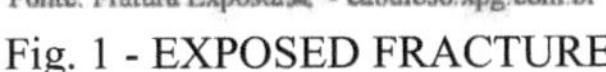

Fonte: Fratura Exposta♔ ~ cabuloso.xpg.com.br

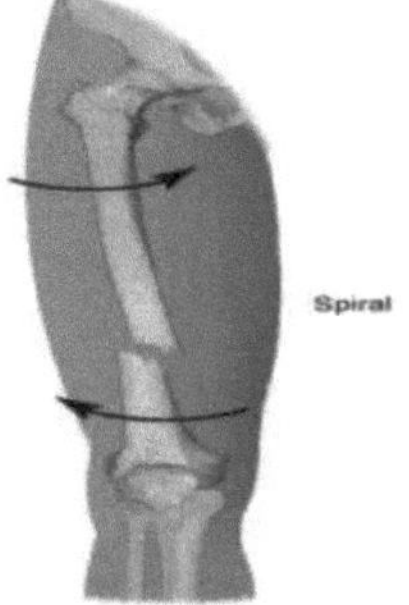

Fonte: o.canbler.com

Fig. 1 - EXPOSED FRACTURE

Fig. 2 - CLOSED FRACTURE

2.4 TREATMENT OBJECTIVES FOR OPEN FRACTURES

The most important objectives in the treatment of open fractures are: (a) to restore function through muscle and joint rehabilitation as early as possible; (b) to prevent infection; (c) to restore soft tissue; and (d) to allow bone healing while avoiding vicious consolidation. Of these objectives, the most important is to prevent infection, because it is the most common event and a determining factor in the occurrence of vicious consolidation, lack of consolidation and loss of function[20] .

2.5 FRACTURE CLASSIFICATION ACCORDING TO GUSTILLO AND ANDERSON

The most widely recognised classification, which to a certain extent is endorsed by clinical practice and the literature, is that proposed by Gustillo and Anderson[21] in 1976. Three types of fracture are identified: those secondary to exposure through the fragment piercing the skin, i.e. low energy (type I); those secondary to low energy external trauma that exposes the bone at the site of the violence, producing limited injury (type II); and the most serious, in which there is extensive exposure, contamination and/or devitalisation (type III). In 1984, Gustillo et al.[22] proposed a subdivision of type III into three subtypes, based on the possibility of wound closure by the skin integument and the presence of vascular damage (Table 1).

A GRADE I open fracture generally consists of a simple, clean fracture with minimal soft tissue injuries and a skin wound smaller than 1 cm. It is a fracture caused by a low-energy injury in which a bone spicule pierces the skin from the inside out, causing a puncture wound. Bacterial contamination is generally very low in these cases, unless the injury occurs in a highly contaminated environment. In grade I fractures, muscle damage is minimal or absent. Of course, a grade I fracture should not be judged by the size of its wound alone, because small wounds can be dangerously contaminated depending on the environment in which they occurred (for example, a fall in a stable).

A GRADE II open fracture consists of a bone lesion with little comminution, a wound larger than 1 cm, with a small soft tissue lesion, but with contamination. These injuries are generally caused from the outside in, with moderate muscle damage. There may be little debris in the fracture site.

A GRADE III open fracture consists of a usually comminuted and deviated bone injury, with exposure of the fracture site, with a wound larger than 10 cm, large comminution, caused by high-energy trauma, with severe soft tissue injuries; loss of a bone segment; fracture associated with vascular injury requiring repair; crushing of muscles, tendons, vessels and/or nerves. This fracture occurs due to high-energy trauma, from the outside in, with a large amount of debris in the fracture site and extensive muscle devitalisation. It is usually deviated or comminuted, although this is not an essential component. There is extensive loss of the skin lining. Fifty per cent of all patients who suffer a grade III injury will end up with functional impairment[23] .

Grade III fractures are subdivided into:

GRADE IIIA: Wound larger than 10 cm with soft tissue kneading and significant contamination, and skin covering of the bone is usually possible.

GRADE IIIB: Wound larger than 10 cm with soft tissue crumpling and contamination, and the skin covering the bone is usually inadequate and requires free or sliding skin flaps.

GRADE IIIC: These are fractures with a wound larger than 10 cm in which there is significant vascular damage, requiring repair to save the limb.

Table 1. Classification of fractures according to Gustillo and Anderson

Type	Wound	Contamination	Soft tissue and bone injuries
I	< 1 cm	Clean	Minimal soft tissue and bone damage
II	1 cm<x<10cm	Moderate	Moderate bone damage
IIIA	> 10 cm	Contaminated	Severe + skin coverage possible
IIIB	> 10 cm	Contaminated	Severe + loss of skin coverage.
IIIC	> 10 cm	Contaminated	Vascular injury requiring repair

Source: Gustillo RB, Anderson JT. Prevention of infection in the treatment of one thousand and twenty-five open fractures of long bones: retrospective and prospective analyses. J *Bone and Joint Surg,* n 58-A, pp. 453 - 458, June 1976.

2.6 CLASSIFICATION OF LESIONS ACCORDING TO TSCHERNE AND OESTERN

Tscheme and Oestem[24] described a classification for fractures with concomitant soft tissue injury, with and without fracture exposure. They pointed out that, despite non-exposure, some fractures behave like open fractures due to the impairment of the soft tissue barrier that separates them from the external environment. Closed fractures were divided into four types (grades 0 to 3) and open fractures into four types (grades 1 to 4). This system is the most widely used in Europe. Its strength is that it considers each component of the soft tissue envelope and valorises soft tissue injury in fractures without exposure.

Tscheme's classification[24] of open fractures stays the involvement of soft tissues in four types: Grade I injuries correspond to closed or open fractures, with little soft tissue contusion, the result of trauma from the inside out. In grade II, there are open injuries resulting from direct trauma with moderate soft tissue contusion, laceration, flictenae and intense oedema, and compartment syndrome may occur. Grade III includes injuries also caused by direct trauma, with intense contusion, crushing, extensive muscle or vascular damage and some degree of compartment syndrome. At the top of the classification are grade IV injuries, in which partial or total amputation and vascular damage requiring repair can occur. As this study only refers to open fractures, only the Tscheme classification[19] was used for open fractures (Table 2).

Table 2. Tscheme and Oestem classification

GRADES	TYPE OF FRACTURE	SOFT TISSUE INJURY	CAUSE
GRADE I	closed or open fractures	little soft tissue contusion	trauma from the inside out.
GRADE II	open fractures	Moderate contusion, laceration, flictenas and intense oedema, possible trauma syndrome compartmental	direct trauma
GRADE III	open fractures	Intensacontusion , crushing, extensive muscle or vascular damage and compartment syndrome to some degree	direct trauma
GRADE IV	open fractures	partial or total amputation,	direct trauma

		vascular damage requiring repair	

Source: Oestem H-J, Tscheme H. Pathophysiology and classification of soft tissue injuries associated with fractures. In: Tscheme H. GotzenL, Eds.fractures with soft tissue injuries. Berlin, etc: Springer-Verlag. 1984: 1-8.

According to Rittmann and Matter[25] , open fractures are accompanied by soft tissue injuries of varying extent. The assessment and treatment of these fractures depends more on the extent and severity of the soft tissue injuries than on the type of fracture.

Depending on the extent of soft tissue damage, three specific consequences can result[26] :

1. Contamination of the wound by bacteria from the external environment;

2. Contusion of soft tissues; crushing, tearing and devascularisation of these tissues, making them more susceptible to bacterial infections;

3. Muscle/bone tearing and/or loss of soft tissues, which normally constitute a sheath for the bone, can affect the methods by which the fracture can be effectively immobilised, and can also deprive the fracture site of the usual contribution of the overlying soft tissues to the bone healing process (generation of progenitor cells for union and healing), as well as there can be direct loss of function due to destroyed muscles, tendons, nerves, vessels and skin.

The extent of soft tissue damage consequently causes[26] :

- Destabilising the fracture;

- Difficulty in consolidation due to deprivation of the bone's nutrient circulation;

- Loss of function (due to damage to the skin, muscles, tendons, nerves and vessels).

While consequence number 1 (contamination by bacteria) is practically universal, the remaining two vary according to "the extent of soft tissue damage". This means that a patient with a small soft tissue injury, properly treated, is of little concern; it has a very different evolution from another with a large soft tissue injury, which may even require immediate amputation.

2.7 PATHOPHYSIOLOGY OF MUSCULOSKELETAL INJURIES

Violent trauma to the musculoskeletal system typically results in extensive ruptures of soft and hard tissues. They can introduce foreign material and bacteria, create ischaemic soft tissue segments, tissue necrosis and empty spaces. The haematoma, contaminated by the foreign material, dissects the tissue planes detached by the trauma, fills the empty spaces and acts as an ideal culture medium for bacteria. Within the first few hours, neutrophils and macrophages enter the wound, with monocytes being found later. Simultaneously, the complement and coagulation systems are activated. Vasoactive substances (serotonin, prostaglandins, kinins, histamine) together with the coagulation system increase vascular permeability. This is followed by massive exudation of plasma proteins and leucocytes[27] .

As for the inflammatory response and tissue repair, the following conditions can occur[27] :

- When the lesion is small, complete debridement is carried out with the removal of bacterial agents and devitalised (necrotic) tissue. In this case, the inflammatory response is controlled and the wound heals.

- When the lesions are massive, with severe contamination or timid intervention, a different result is observed. The macrophages are unable to cope with the bacterial load; they die and release lysosomal or proteolytic enzymes, causing necrosis of the surrounding tissues. Necrosis associated with increased tissue pressure forms a vicious circle with progressive inflammation, muscle ischaemia, compartment syndromes, tissue loss and spreading infection. The progressive inflammatory response is most often seen after contamination of an open fracture, but can also occur in closed fractures and dislocations or after simple crushing of muscle compartments.

2.8 PROGNOSIS OF OPEN FRACTURES

The prognosis of open fractures is mainly determined by the amount of devitalised soft tissue caused by the injury and the type of bacterial contamination. These two factors working in combination, rather than the configuration of the fracture itself, are the main determinants of the outcome[20] .

The extent of soft tissue devitalisation is determined by the energy absorbed by the limb at the time of injury. The most important and ultimate goal in the treatment of open fractures is to restore the function of the patient's limb as early and completely as possible. To achieve this goal, the surgeon must prevent infection, restore soft tissues, achieve bone union, avoid vicious consolidation, and institute early joint movement and muscle rehabilitation. Of these objectives, the most important is to avoid infection, because it is the most common event and a determining factor in the occurrence of vicious consolidation, lack of consolidation and loss of function[20 ,28] .

2.9 COMPLICATIONS OF OPEN FRACTURES

1. OSTEOMYELITIS: taking care of the soft tissues and using stable fixation allows the fracture to heal and reduces the risk of infection.

2. PSEUDOARTHROSIS: more common in open fractures, those with marked displacement or inefficient fixation.

3. VICIOUS CONSOLIDATION: may require osteotomy to correct the deformity.

4. COMPARTIMENTAL SYNDROME: may require immediate intervention such as fasciotomy.

One of the most dreaded complications of surgical treatment is post-operative infection, which significantly increases the cost and duration of treatment and jeopardises functional results and long-term rehabilitation, thus representing a challenge for the orthopaedic surgeon.

The main risk factors for post-operative fracture infection are[5] :

1. Degree of energy of the trauma;
2. Degree of soft tissue injuries;
3. Degree of local contamination;
4. Osteosynthesis surgical time;
5. The patient's immunological status.

Often the infectious process sets in before the fracture has healed, which makes treatment even more difficult[29] . The risk of infection after an open fracture depends on the degree of contamination and the amount of devitalised tissue[6] . Recently, other patient-related factors, such as immunological status and smoking, have also been identified as risk factors for the development of infection[11] . Studies in large series show infection rates of less than 1% for closed fractures and rates of between 2.4% and 4.8% for open fractures[30 ,31] .

In open fractures, some factors are decisive for the onset of infection: exposure time, the amount of soft tissue (directly related to the kinetic energy absorbed) and the degree of tissue devitalisation, which not only make coverage procedures more difficult, but can also alter the vitality of the bone and the repair process[3] .

Currently, open fractures are treated with the following initial objectives: to prevent infection, to promote the restoration of soft tissues and to fix the fracture with adequate alignment and sufficient stability for the patient's comfort, as well as to allow dressings and other procedures to be carried out.

Knowing the characteristics of the trauma can give the surgeon an idea of the degree of tissue destruction and necrosis, while always remembering that the same kinetic energy absorbed by the bone is also distributed to the soft tissues.

The time between the fracture and hospitalisation is also crucial. Up to the point of 6 to 8 hours, the wound can be considered contaminated. After this period, the contaminating bacteria may already be in the process of multiplying and spreading through the tissues, thus characterising a situation of infection[3] .

From a historical point of view, the basic work that gave rise to the principle of emergency treatment for open fractures was carried out in 1988, the landmark experiment by Freidrich[32] , in which bacterial replication rates were assessed in a wound caused to guinea pigs (Cavia *porcellus),* reaching the conclusion that high rates of cell division were detected after 6 hours. In this line of thought, the so-called "Six hour rule" was developed, according to which this period would be a determining factor in the difference between contaminated tissue and an actual infection. It is important to remember, however, that the percentage of infections is 10 to 20 times higher than in closed fractures.

2.10 BONE INFECTION (OSTEOMYELITIS)

Bone infection is known worldwide as osteomyelitis. It is an infection characterised by progressive destruction of the cortical bone and medullary cavity[33] .

Osteomyelitis has been classified in various ways, taking into account certain criteria, such as the location of the process, the extent of bone involvement, the host's immunological status, comorbidities and the type of causative agent[33,34] .

Post-traumatic osteomyelitis results from direct inoculation of the microorganism into the bone and surrounding areas at the time of the trauma. There is also contamination by intra-hospital agents resulting from peri- or post-operative manipulation[33] .

Chart 3. Risk of infection in open fractures. Gustillo 1988.

TYPE OF FRACTURE	RISK OF INFECTION
Type I	Up to 2%
Type II	2-7%
Type IIIA	7%
Type IIIB	10-50%
Type III C	25 - 50%

Source: Gustillo apud Lima and Zumiotti,
[27] http://www.praticahospitalar.com.br/pratica%2052/pdfs/mat%2001.pdf.
Accessed on: 24 January 2013.

In a prospective study of 134 patients with open fractures of the lower limbs of types II, IIIA, IIIB, IIIC of the Gustillo classification, treated at the Institute of Orthopaedics and Traumatology of the Hospital das Clínicas of the Faculty of Medicine of the University of São Paulo (IOT) in 2000 and 2001, the following predisposing factors to osteomyelitis were observed in the evolution of the treatment of open fractures: patient severity (ASA classification), fractures of the femur and associated bones, wound kept open after initial debridement and immediate internal fixation[33] .

The aetiological agents that predominate in exposed post-traumatic infections are *Staphylococcus aureus* and a variety of gram-negative bacilli that vary according to the local hospital microbiota. The association of aetiological agents in the same patient is not uncommon. Infections are therefore a complication of open fractures, and the most common germs causing these bone infections are streptococci and staphylococci.

Patients most often present with fever, local inflammatory signs and purulent secretion draining from the surgical wound or wound that is still exposed.

CHAPTER 3

OBJECTIVES

- To identify the risk factors associated with infection in patients with open fractures;
- Create a score to enable risk stratification during initial care.

CHAPTER 4

PATIENTS AND METHODS

A retrospective study based on medical records was carried out between March and December 2009, with the target population being patients diagnosed with open fractures treated at the Roberto Santos General Hospital (HGRS) in Salvador-Bahia. The research project was submitted to the Research Ethics Committee (CEP) of the Bahiana School of Medicine and Public Health (EBMS), where it was approved under protocol number[2] 121/2009.

The study included all hospitalised patients over the age of 8, of both sexes, with an open fracture, admitted via the HGRS emergency department or from other hospitals in the public health system in the state of Bahia, who arrived at the HGRS Orthopaedic Service via the State Patient Regulation Centre (CER). Patients with open fractures of the axial skeleton (face, skull, thorax) and those who did not remain in the hospital for at least one day after the initial procedure, either due to death or transfer, were excluded from the study.

The HGRS is the largest public hospital in the Northeast of Brazil and serves the population of the city of Salvador (capital of Bahia) and the entire interior of the state through the CER (State Reference Centre), being responsible for assisting a population of approximately 14 million people and an area of around 565,000 km. The HGRS Orthopaedic Service is structured to treat open and closed fractures and specialises in this type of care. Initial care involves filling in a standardised clinical form for assessing orthopaedic patients, which remains attached to the medical records. This form is updated throughout the hospitalisation period and compiles clinical and demographic data, as well as the main events concerning the patient, including the presence or absence of infection. The existence of this medical record made the study possible and all the data used to carry out the research was extracted from it.

The independent variables used for analysis were age, gender, marital status (single, married, other), place of origin (capital or interior of the state of Bahia), bone affected (upper limbs and lower limbs), type of accident (traffic - motorcycling, car driving and being run over; PAF - firearm perforation; trauma - falling from a height, direct trauma), fracture exposure time (time elapsed between the trauma and the therapeutic approach), fracture classifications according to Gustillo *et al?* classification of soft tissue injuries according to Tscheme and Oestem[24] , as well as habits such as drinking and smoking. The outcome infection was adopted as the dependent variable.

Infection (outcome variable) was identified based on clinical and laboratory findings, according to the criteria for early infection within a two-week period proposed by Willenegger[35] .

This means that an infected lesion was considered to be a wound that showed any aspect of superficial or deep infection associated or not with fever, leucocytosis and elevated erythrocyte sedimentation rate (ESR)[35,36] . To verify this outcome, patients were assessed during hospitalisation and after two weeks of follow-up, regardless of discharge.

During the period adopted for the study, it was possible to collect data from 122 medical records that met the inclusion criteria and whose clinical records were filled in acceptably. Of this total, the outcome infection (dependent variable) was confirmed in 31 patients, 91 of whom were free of infection. In order to analyse the risk factors associated with infection, the study participants were divided into two groups: patients with and without infection.

The data was presented in frequency distribution tables for discrete variables and as mean and standard deviation for continuous variables. To analyse the risk factors associated with infection, the two groups (with and without infection) were compared using the chi-square test for discrete variables and Student's *t-test* for continuous variables. The value of $p < 0.05$ was adopted as the significance level for all tests.

Taking into account the statistical significance found in the bivariate analysis and in order to select variables that predict infection, a multivariate analysis was carried out. Based on the final logistic regression model, the *Odds-Ratio of* each variable was calculated. Based on the identification of variables significantly associated with infection in the bivariate and multivariate analyses, a score was devised to predict the risk of this outcome at the time of initial patient care.

To construct the score, called the Infection Risk Score (IRS), relevant factors were selected (statistically and clinically), i.e. those considered predictors of infection. Thus, three variables were included in the ERI, namely the Tscheme[24] and Gustillo[22] classifications, as well as the fracture exposure time. With regard to exposure time, there was a need to redistribute it into three categories, i.e. up to 12 hours of exposure, 12 to 24 hours of exposure and over 24 hours. This subdivision was made to transform time into a categorical variable and was based on the study by Patzakis and Wilkins[37] .

The score was developed as follows: for exposure time, scores of 1 (exposure time of up to 12 hours), 2 (exposure time of 12 to 24 hours) and 3 (exposure time of more than 24 hours) were considered; for the Gustillo classification[17] , scores of 1 for type I (mild), 2 for type II (moderate), 3 for type IIIA (severe A), and 5 for type IIIC (severe C) were considered. (severe A), score 4 for type IIIB (severe B) and score 5 for type IIIC (severe C); and, for the Tscheme classification[24] , score 1 for type I, score 2 for type II, score 3 for type III and 4 for type IV. These variables were then transformed into a sum of the individual scores for each patient. This data made it possible to construct the ERI, which ranged from 3 for the lowest risk of infection to 12 for the highest risk of infection (Figure 3).

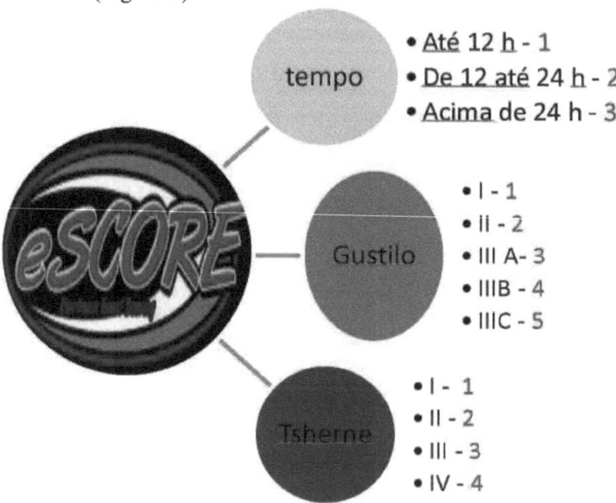

Figura 3. Demonstration of the formation of the ERI score

Next, in order to identify the association between the ERI and the outcome of infection, the Student's *t-test* was used for the association between the median score in the two groups and the qualitative variable infection. The ERI was also categorised into three levels to identify the risk of infection: Level I (low risk) - patients with 3, 4 and 5 points on the ERI; Level II (intermediate risk) - patients with 6, 7, 8 and 9 points on the ERI; Level III (high risk) - patients with 10, 11 and 12 points on the ERI (Figure 4).

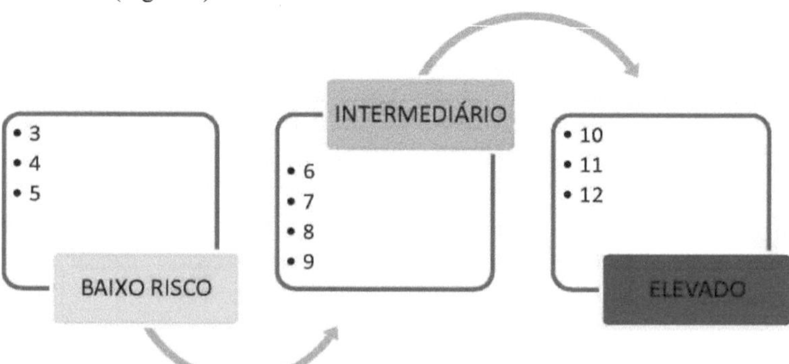

Figura 4. ERI x Severity levels

CHAPTER 5

RESULTS

The total study sample comprised 122 participants (Table 1). Of this total, the distribution by gender revealed that more men were affected (83.6%) than women (16.4%). The overall infection rate was 25.4% (31 patients). The average age was 31.5 (± 13.5) years in the group with infection and 31.7 (±14.3) in the group without infection. Most of the sample consisted of single individuals (64.2%), with a high prevalence of drinking (67.2%) and smoking (38.5%). The lower limbs were more affected (63.9%) than the upper limbs (36.1%). The most frequent type of accident in the sample was traffic-related (45.1%). Patients came predominantly from the state capital in the group without infection (61.1%) and from the countryside in the group with infection (61.3%).

Table 1. Sociodemographic data of patients with open fractures in a public hospital in the state of Bahia between March and December 2009.

Variable	With infection	No infection	Total N	p-value
Sex	31	91	122	0,963
Male	26 (83,9%)	76 (83,5%)	102(83,6%)	
Female	5 (16,1%)	15 (16,5%)	20(16,4%)	
Marital status	26	83	109	0,773
Single	15 (57,7%)	55 (66,3%)	70(64,2%)	
Married	10 (38,5%)	25 (30,1%)	35(32,1%)	
Others	1 (3,8%)	3 (3,6%)	4(3,7%)	
Origin	31	90	121	0,080
Capital	12 (38,7%)	55(61,1%)	67(55,4%)	
Inside	19(61,3%)	35 (38,9%)	54(44,6%)	
Location	31	91	122	0,345
MMII	22 (71,0%)	56(61,5%)	78(63,9%)	
MMSS	9 (29,0%)	35(38,5%)	44(36,1%)	
Type of trauma	31	91	122	0,138
PAF	5(16,1%)	29(31,9%)	34(27,9%)	
Trauma	10(32,2%)	23(25,3%)	33(27,0%)	
Transit	16(51,6%)	39(42,8%)	55(45,1%)	
Smoking	31	91	122	0,687
Smokers	11(35,5%)	36(39,6%)	47(38,5%)	
Alcoholism	31	91	122	0,942
Alcoholics	21(67,7%)	61(67,0%)	82(67,2%)	

In terms of sociodemographic characteristics, no association was found between infection and marital status, gender, location of the affected limb, type of trauma, lifestyle habits or the patient's origin (Table 1). No association was found between infection and anthropometric measurements such as weight, age and BMI, although there was a significant difference in the height variable (Table 2).

Table 2. Anthropometric profile of patients with open fractures in a public hospital in the state of Bahia between March and December 2009.

Variable	With infection	No infection	Total N	p-value
Age	31,5 (±13,5)	31,7 (±14,3)	118	0,929
Weight	71,9 (±14,2)	67,9 (±14,1)	89	0,269

| Height | 1,76 (± 0,1) | 1,71 (±0,1) | 84 | 0,036 |
| BMI | 23,5 (± 3,0) | 22,8 (± 6,1) | 53 | 0,669 |

As for the clinical conditions assessed, all showed a significant association. Fracture exposure time (between the accident and the start of surgical treatment) averaged 30.3 hours (± 19.5%) for the group with infection and 21.4 hours (± 12.1%) for the group without infection. The earliest approach was 6 hours after the trauma, and the latest 76 hours after the accident. The occurrence of infection was significantly associated with exposure time. According to the Gustillo classification[22] , type III fractures (74.2%) were more likely to be infected than the other types. According to the Tscheme classification[24] , type III (48.4%) and II (25.8%) injuries were the ones with the highest risk of developing infection (Table 3).

Table 3. Clinical characteristics of open fractures in a public hospital in the state of Bahia between March and December 2009.

Variable	With infection	No infection	Total N	p-value
Exposure time Hours	25	79	94	0,007
	30,3 h (±19,5)	21,4 h (±12,1)		
Gustillo	31	91	122	0,042
I	1 (3,2%)	10(11,0%)	11	
II	7 (22,6%)	39 (42,8%)	46	
IIIA	7 (22,6%)	20 (22,0%)	27	
IIIB	13 (41,9%)	19 (20,9%)	32	
IIIC	3 (9,7%)	3 (3,3%)	06	
Tscheme	31	91	122	0,001
I	6(19,4%)	32 (35,2%)	38	
II	8 (25,8%)	43 (47,2%)	51	
III	15 (48,4%)	15(16,5%)	30	
IV	2 (6,5%)	1 (14%)	03	

The multivariate analysis was carried out and the *Odds Ratio* values were found for the variables that showed statistical significance in the bivariate analysis (Table 4).

Table *O* - *Odds-ratio* for each variable

variables	B	S.E.	Wald	df	Sig.	Exp(B)	95% C.I.for EXP(B) Lower	Upper
Time	,040	,017	5,556	1	,018	1,041	1,007	1,076
Gustillo	,284	,304	,869	1	,351	1,328	,731	2,411
Tscherne	,641	,408	2,468	1	,116	1,899	,853	4,225
Constant	-4,413	1,014	18,953	1	,000	,012		

However, bivariate analysis was used to calculate the score, since the logistic regression model carried out in enter and backwald mode only found statistical significance in the time variable.

The Infection Risk Score (IRS) had a mean of 7.12 for the total group of patients. When the ERI averages were compared between the groups - with infection (8.24) and without infection (6.77), it was possible to see a statistically significant difference with p=0.001 (Figure 5).

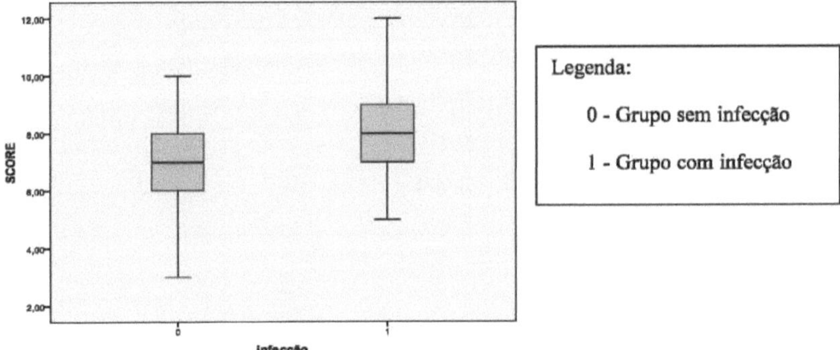

Figura 5. *Boxplot* graph showing the comparison of the median scores of the groups with and without infection.

The ROC curve (Figure 6), constructed from the ERI, showed a direct relationship between the ERI and the infection outcome, with the area under the curve estimated at 0.709 (p= 0.002), a result considered satisfactory for assessing association in clinical studies[38] . The accuracy of the ERI can be assessed from the characteristics of the curve at the cut-off point selected for the outcome, which was 6.5. At this point, the curve's accuracy parameters are sensitivity of 0.840 and specificity of 0.544 (Chart 4).

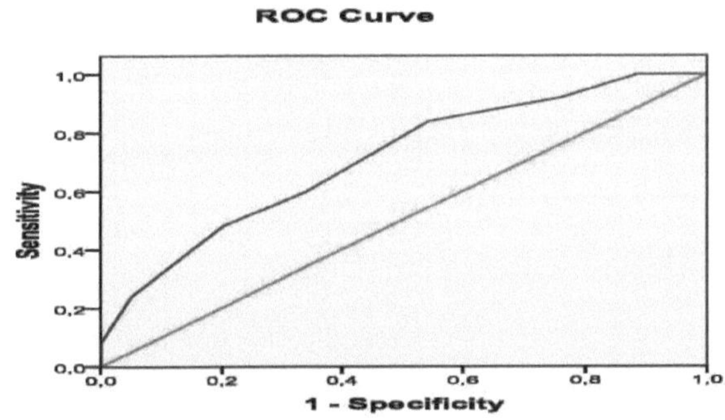

Figura 6. ROC curve

Table 4. Sensitivity and specificity of the SPSS ROC curve

Cut-off points	Sensitivity	1 - Specificity
2,0000	1,000	1,000
3,5000	1,000	0,987
4,5000	1,000	0,886

5,5000	0,920	0,759
6,5000	0,840	0,544
7,5000	0,600	0,342
8,5000	0,480	0,203
9,5000	0,240	0,051
11,0000	0,080	0,000
13,0000	0,000	0,000

CHAPTER 6

DISCUSSION

The results of this study reveal that the clinical factors that were significantly associated with infection in the final outcome were the time elapsed since the accident, the type of open fracture according to Gustillo[22] and the type of soft tissue injury according to Tscheme[24] . These three variables were used to design the ERI, resulting in a score that is capable of predicting the risk of infection from an open fracture at the time of the patient's first assessment. The ERI had a sensitivity of 0.84 and specificity of 0.55, with a cut-off point of 6.5. The area under the ROC curve was also considered satisfactory for the clinical assessment parameters (0.709)[38] .

Although most of the sociodemographic and anthropometric variables were not significantly associated with infection, the evaluation of these variables added important data on the profile of the population assisted. The overall infection rate was 25.4 per cent, with a predominance of males (83.6 per cent), a prevalence of single individuals (64.2 per cent), with an average age of 31.5 years; the lower limbs were the most commonly involved (63.9 per cent), and traffic accidents accounted for 45.1 per cent of all patients in the sample. There was also a high prevalence of alcohol use (67.2%) and smoking (38.5%).

The sociodemographic data in this study is in line with the results of several previous reports on the subject. Spencer *et al?* found a mean age of 45 years and 40% of the sample had been involved in road traffic accidents. Chua et al.[39] found an average age of 36.5 years, 91.3% of patients were male, and 69% had been involved in road traffic accidents. Miiller et *al?* and Moore et *al?* also found that the majority of their patients were male, with a mean age of 35.2 and 31 years, respectively. As for the type of trauma, Moore et *al.* found 52 per cent were road traffic accidents and Miiller et *al.* found a prevalence of 38.4 per cent. Even though this type of trauma is not identified as a factor associated with infection, there is evidence of the considerable frequency of this type of high-energy trauma, resulting in more complex open fractures with a greater chance of infection as a final outcome.

Bowen and Widmaier[11] showed that tobacco use and the patient's immunological status were risk factors for developing an infection. In our study, although the number of patients using alcohol and tobacco was high, this association was not confirmed. In a similar study, Pollak et al.[10] found an association between smoking and infection. However, the high prevalence of alcohol use that we found reinforces the study by Arruda et al.[40] , who found a strong association between road traffic accidents and the use of alcohol and illicit drugs before the trauma.

The overall infection rate in this study is higher than the rates reported in previous studies. Kamat et al.[41] found an infection rate of 11.6 per cent, Singh et *al.*[42] found 14.9 per cent, and Spencer et *al?* showed 14.6 per cent of infection cases. Some differences in these studies can be pointed out in comparison with our findings. In Kamat's study there were only 21.3% of Gustillo type III fractures[22] and all cases were operated on in less than 17 hours; 93% of patients with Gustillo type III injuries[22] (49.5%) in Spencer's study were treated within 12 hours; and 69% of Gustillo type III fractures were treated within 6 hours in Singh's study.

On the other hand, the study by Pollak et al.[10] showed 27% of infected fractures, which is very similar to our rate (25.4%). All the fractures in this study were Gustillo type III[22] and were produced by high-energy trauma, and 41.7% of the patients were treated within 10 hours of the trauma. Our study consisted of 53.3% Gustillo type III fractures[22] and debridement took an average of 30.3 hours for the infection group and 21.4 hours for the non-infection group. We believe that this higher infection rate can be explained by both the severity of the cases and the delay in treatment. Individuals from other cities were more likely to develop an infection than those from the state capital. It's possible that the individuals were referred to the capital due to the lack of hospital units or suitable treatment facilities, especially for the most serious cases.

The Gustillo[22] and Tscheme[24] classifications were shown in this study to be important predictors of infection. This agrees with the majority of studies regarding the Gustillo classification, but there are few studies evaluating the participation of the Tscheme classification as a predictor of infection. Gustillo[43] , in his 1989 study, presented a 0% infection rate for type I fractures, 2.5% for type II, 13.7% for type IIIA, 5% for type IIIB and 44.4% for type IIIC. Miiller et al. found an infection rate of 68.8 per cent for Gustillo type III for an exposure time of more than 6 hours. Recently, Chua et al.[39] showed an infection rate of 8.5 per cent for Gustillo type I[22] , 9.4 per cent for type II, 21.8 per cent for type IIIA, and 44.6 per cent for types IIIB and IIIC. The lesions most strongly associated with infection found in our study, in relation to Tscheme's classification of soft tissue lesions, were those of types II and III. These results also agree with Miiller *et al.*[3] who found a high infection rate in type III and IV lesions of the Tscheme classification.

Although the correlation between time and infection is not a consensus in orthopaedic literature, there is evidence of its strength. Spencer et al.[9] , Kamat et al.[41] , and Singh et al.[42] found no association between infection and time to first debridement. On the other hand, in our study, this variable proved to be an important predictor of infection in open fractures. Kindsfater and Jonassen[44] carried out a comparative study of tibial fractures, Gustillo types II and III[22] , in which there were no statistically different results with osteomyelitis in the groups operated on before and 5 hours after the trauma (7% and 38%, respectively). In the study by Pollak et al.[10] , infection was not associated with delay in debridement, but time from injury to hospital admission was a predictor of infection, considering time as a continuous variable. In the same study, considering time as a categorical variable, there was a significant chance of infection when hospitalisation lasted longer than 2 hours (5.4 times more likely to have an infection) and the risk of infection was significantly higher when patients were transferred to the trauma centre 11 hours after the injury.

All these previous studies presented time as a categorical variable divided into multiples of five or six hours. In addition, only a few fractures were treated after 12 hours, for example only 8 (7%) in the study by Spencer et *al?* In our study, time was also used as a categorical variable. Thus, we used multiple 12-hour intervals, similar to the model adopted by Patzakis and Wilkins[37] . This division was used because none of the fractures were treated in less than 6 hours of exposure, most being treated after 12 hours. Therefore, we believe that the time of injury measured as a categorical variable is a significant predictor when the delay is greater than 12 hours, and may help to elucidate some of the previous results in the orthopaedic literature.

Although orthopaedic surgeons agree that preventing infection is a crucial issue in the treatment of open fractures, few studies have been dedicated to evaluating predictive factors in these cases. Our study not only analysed the factors associated with infection, but also identified those that were combined with a stronger association with infection to construct the so-called ERI score. This score was satisfactory in its objectives and especially adequate in terms of its sensitivity to infection (84 per cent). No similar results were found in the literature, although much emphasis has been placed on individual variables associated with infection, especially the time elapsed between the accident and effective treatment, and the severity of the injury according to Gustillo[22] .

The basic purpose of the ERI is to provide a useful tool for predicting the risk of infection in open fractures at the time of the patient's admission to the emergency room, given that all the variables used for the ERI are collected from the results required in the initial clinical assessment. The ERI could therefore guide the orthopaedic surgeon in the first surgical approach, which would be as aggressive as necessary according to the risk of infection. Factors such as extent of debridement, primary closure of the lesion, type and timing of antibiotics, type of fracture fixation could be decided on the basis of the ERI. Post-operative therapy, nursing care and patient rehabilitation can also be selected according to the ERI score.

CHAPTER 7

LIMITATIONS AND PROSPECTS

This work was carried out using information from medical records, which was not always complete, making it impossible to carry out some analyses that could have complemented the study. Or rather, some medical records lacked data on smoking, alcohol consumption, previous illnesses, in short, data to carry out analyses that could add more concise results to the study.

In addition, some statistical sub-analyses may have been distorted since the sample size effect was used specifically for the infection outcome.

The final categorisation of the score (ERI) into severity levels I, II, III - mild, moderate and severe, respectively - takes on a conservative profile, with score 6 being considered moderate, 3,4,5 as mild and 10,11 and 12 as severe.

When creating the score, time was also a limiting factor, as exposure time was categorised subjectively; we tried to categorise time as homogeneously as possible, as no delimiting elements had been identified in previous studies. Thus, multiple times of 12 were assumed due to the hypothesised direct relationship between exposure time and patient infection.

Aspects related to other infection indicators, as well as the strength of the association between these factors, still need to be studied in greater depth so that their true role as a guide to behaviour can be properly assessed.

There is a need for further research into the relationship between risk factors and infection in open fractures, with a larger sample size and data from multiple centres, so that other studies can complement and confirm the knowledge built up in this study.

CHAPTER 8

CONCLUSION

This article provides the literature with several original contributions on the subject. Our data reinforces the association between infection and the variables exposure time and injury severity in open fractures. Gustillo's classification[22] had already been used several times in the literature, but our study is one of the few that has used Tscheme's classification[24] , thus demonstrating its strongest association among all the factors. A risk score (RRI) was created to predict infection, which can be used in the initial approach to the patient with 0.840 specificity and 0.544 sensitivity. It can also make an important contribution so that it can be used in future studies that take its validation into account.

CHAPTER 9

BIBLIOGRAPHICAL REFERENCES

1. Ashford RU, Mehta JA, Cripps R: Delayed presentation is no barrier to satisfactory outcome in the management of open tibial fractures. Injury. 2004, 35:411-416.

2. Harley BJ, Beaupre LA, Jones CA, et al. The effect of time to definitive treatment on the rate of nonunion and infection in open fractures. J Orthop Traum. 2002, 16:484-490.

4. Miiller SS, Sadenberg T, Pereira GJC, et al. Epidemiological, clinicai and microbiological prospective study of patients with open fractures assisted at a university hospital. Acta Ortop Bras. 2003,11:158-169.

5. Silva AGP, Silva FBA, Santos ALG, et al. Infection after intramedullary stabilisation of diaphyseal fractures of the lower limbs: treatment protocol. Acta Ortop Bras. 2008, 16(5): 266-269.

6. Cleveland KB. Infection: General principles. In Canale ST. Campbell's orthopaedic surgery. Translation by Maurício Kfuri Júnior. lOTh Ed. São Paulo: Manole. 2006, 643-659.

7. Moore TJ, Mauney C, Barron J. The uses of quantitative bacterial counts in open fractures. Clin Orthop Relat Res. 1989, 248:227-230.

8. Khatod M, Botte MJ, Hoyt DB, et al. Outcomes in open tibia fractures: relationship between delay in treatment and infection. J Trauma. 2003, 55: 949-954.

9. Skaggs DL, Friend L, Alman B, et al. The effect of surgical delay on acute infection following 554 open fractures in children. J Bone Joint Surg Am. 2005, 87: 8-12.

10. Spencer J, Smith A, Woods D. The effect of time delay on infection in open long-bone fractures: a 5-year prospective audit from a district general hospital. Ann R Coll Surg Eng. 2004, 86:108-112.

11. Pollak AN, Jones AL, Castillo RC, et al. The Relationship Between Time to Surgical Debridement and Incidence of Infection After Open High-Energy Lower Extremity Trauma. J Bone Joint Surg Am. 2012, 92:7-15.

12. Bowen TR, Widmaier JC. Hast classification predicts infection after open fracture. Clin Orthop Relat Res. 2005, 433:205-211.

13. Lima ALLM, Zumiotti AV, Uip DE, et al. Predictive factors of infection in patients with open fractures of the lower limbs. Acta Ortop Bras. 2004, 12(1).

14. Salter RB. Disorders and injuries of the musculoskeletal system. 2ª. Edition. Publisher: MEDSI. Rio de Janeiro-RJ, 1985.

15. Chiara O, Cimbanassi S. Protocol for in-hospital care of severe trauma. Iª. Edition. Publisher: Elsevier. Rio de Janeiro-RJ, 2009.

16. Thomson A, Skinner A and Piercy J. Tidy's Physiotherapy. Iª. Edition. Editora Livraria Santos.

São Paulo - SP, 1994.

17. Lourenço PRB, Franco JS. Update on the treatment of open fractures. Rev Bras de Ortopedia. 1998, 33(6): 436-446.

18. Paccola CAJ. Open fractures: an update article. Rev Bras de Ortopedia. 2001, 36: 283-291.

19. Lloyd GER. Hippocratic Writings. New York: Pelican Books. 1978, 277-314.

20. Sudkamp NP. Soft tissue injury: Pathophysiology and its influence on fracture management. Ed. Ruedi, TP, Murphy, WM Thieme. 2000, 59.

21. Chapman MW, Olson SA. Open fractures, in Rockwood and Green's fractures in adults - Edited by CA Rockwood, Jr. DP Green, RW Bucholz, JD Heckman 4th edition, v.l, 305-352. Philadelphia: Lippincott-Raven, 1996.

22. Gustillo RB, Anderson JT. Prevention of infection in the treatment of one thousand and twenty-five open fractures of long bones: retrospective and prospective analyses. J Bone and Joint Surg. 1976, 58:453-458.

23. Gustillo RB, Mendonza RM, Williams DN. Problems in the management of type III open fractures: a new classification of type III open fractures. J Trauma. 1984, 24: 742-746.

24. Howard, S. An. Orthopaedic Resident's Manual. Publisher: Revinter Ltda. Rio de Janeiro-RJ, 1995.

25. Oestem HJ, Tscheme H. Pathophysiology and classification of soft tissue injuries associated with fractures. In: Tscheme H. Gotzen L, Eds. fractures with soft tissue injuries. Berlin: Springer-Verlag. 1984, 1-8.

26. Rittmann WW, Matter P. The Exposed Fracture. Ed. Manole Ltda. São Paulo-SP. 1978.

27. Hebert S, Xavier R. Orthopaedics and Traumatology: Principles and Practice. 3ª . Edition. Artmed Publishing House. São Paulo - SP. 2003, 1441-1457.

28. Brown, DE et al. Secrets in Orthopaedics. Artes Médicas. Porto Alegre. 1996.

29. Ottolenghi CE. Exposed fractures. Ed. Universitario de Buenos Aires. Buenos Aires, 1978.

30. Klemm K, Henry S, Seligson D. The treatment of infection after interlocking nailing. Tech Orthop. 1988, 3: 54-61.

31. Sojbjerb JO, Eiskjaer S, Moller-Larsen F. Locked nailing of comminuted and unstable fractures of the femur. J Bone Joint Surg Br. 1990, 72: 23-25.

32. Tometta P, Tiburzi D. Antegrade or retrograde reamed femoral nailing. A prospective, randomised Trial. J Bone Joint Surg Br. 2000, 82: 652-654.

33. Freidrich PL. Die aseptische Versorgung frischer Wundem. Arch Klin Chir. 1898, 57: 288-310.

34. Lima ALLM, Zumiotti AV. Osteomyelitis: a multiprofessional challenge. Infectology. Hospital

Practice. 2007, 11-12.

35.   Lima ALLM, Zumiotti AV. Current aspects of the diagnosis and treatment of osteomyelitis. Acta Ortop Bras. 1999, 7(3): 135-141.

36.   Willenegger H, Roth B. Treatment tactis and late results in early infection following osteosynthesis. Unfallchirurgier. 1986, 12(5): 241-246.

37.   Gamer JS. CDC guideline for prevention of surgical wound infection. Infect Control. 1985, 7:190-200.

38.   Patzakis MJ, Wilkins J. Factors influencing infection rate in open fracture wounds. Clin Orthop. 1989, 243: 36-40.

39.   Website: www.paulomargotto.com.br. ROC curve: How to make and interpret it in SPSS. Accessed 03 Dec 2012.

40.   Chua W, Murphy D, Siow W, et al. Epidemiological analysis of outcomes in 323 open tibial diaphyseal fractures: a nine-year experience. Singapore M Original Article ed J. 2012, 53(6): 385.

41.   Arruda LRP, Silva MAC, Malerba FG, et al. Open fractures: epidemiological and descriptive study. Acta Ortopédica Brasileira. 2009, 17(6): 326-330.

42.   Kamat AS. Infection Rates in Open Fractures of the Tibia: Is the 6-Hour Rule Fact or Fiction? Orthop Adv. 2011.

43.   Singh J, Rambani R, Hashim Z, et al. The relationship between time to surgical debridement and incidence of infection in grade III open fractures. Strategies Trauma Limb Reconstr. 2012, 7(1): 33-37.

44.   Gustilo R.D. Management of open fractures in orthopeadic infection. In: Diagnoses and treatment. Philadelphia: Saunders. 1989, 87-117.

45.   Kindsfater K, Jonassen EA. Osteomyelitis in grade II and III open tibia fractures with late debridement. J Orthop Trauma. 1995, 9: 121-127.

CHAPTER 10

ANNEXES

ANNEX 1 - Roberto Santos General Hospital evaluation form
(used for data collection)

REMARKS: ____

LEITO: _______

NAME: _______

DATE:	ADMISSION:	REGISTRATION:	
LAUDO:		SEX:	
CIVIL STATUS:		NATURALITY:	
DATE OF BIRTH:		PROVINCE:	
WEIGHT:		HEIGHT:	
TRAUMA		SURGERY	
DATE:	TIME:	DATE:	TIME:
TSCHERNE 1:	GUSTILLO 1:	TSCHERNE 2:	GUSTILLO 2:
TYPE OF ACCIDENT: ( ) DOMESTIC TRAFFIC ( ) RUN OVER ( ) MOTORBIKES	( ) PAF ( ) RURAL ( ) SPORT ( ) FALL ( )DIRECT TRAUMA MO ( ) VEHICLE COLLISION	,	( )
INITIAL TREATMENT: ( ) SURGICAL CLEANING ( ) FIXATION			
FIXATION: ( ) EXTERNAL ( ) INTERNAL ( ) TRANSARTICULAR ( ) HYBRID SCREW ( ) MINIMUM		,	( ) ROD ( ) PLATE /
COMPARTMENTAL SYNDROME COMPARTMENT SYNDROME: ( )PRESENT ( ) ABSENT ( ) POSSIBLE			
SUTURE: ( ) PRIMARY ( ) OPEN			
CO-MORBIDITIES: ( ) SMOKING ( ) HTA ( ) DM ( ) ALCOHOLISM			
DIAGNOSIS (FRACTURE)		EXPOSED/CLOSED	CLASSIFICATION
1.			
2.			
3.			

*Medical record

Edit Account | Instructions & Forms | Log Out | Get Help Now

International Orthopaedics Springer SCHOLARONE™ Manuscripts

Main Menu → Author Dashboard → Submission Confirmation

You are logged in as Marcos Matos

Submission Confirmation

Thank you for submitting your manuscript to *International Orthopaedics*.

Manuscript ID: IO-07-13-1033

Title: PREDISPOSING FACTORS FOR INFECTION IN PATIENTS WITH OPEN FRACTURES AND THE PROPOSAL OF A RISK SCORE.

Authors: Matos, Marcos
Lima, Lucynara
Oliveira, Rafael
Oliveira, Luiz

Date Submitted: 02-Jul-2013

Print Return to Dashboard

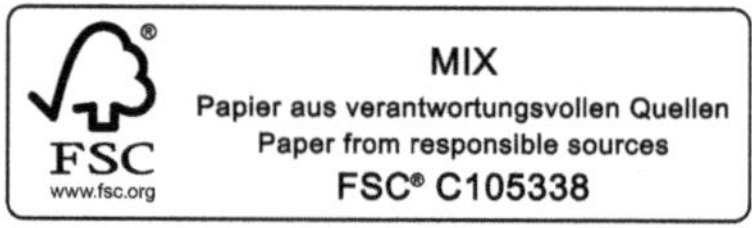

Printed by Books on Demand GmbH, Norderstedt / Germany